Wake Pray Train

Wake Pray Train

Glorifying God With Your Fitness

Robert L. Wagner

P.H.A.T.B.O.Y. Music and Publishing
Arlington, Texas

To Miracle for your patience as I have spent resources and time training, competing, and helping others. Your support constantly amazes me.

To the many influencers (i.e. Pastors, Fellow Trainers, Friends, etc) who have encouraged, educated, or challenged me. I salute you all.

To the many Fit Christians (i.e. supporters) around the globe that have supported the movement from the inception; every hashtag, shirt purchase, or Like/Comment/Share has been beneficial to the growth of this.

Contents

INTRODUCTION

When I was a freshman in college, I was rocked by the grace of God. Although I grew up in a spiritually active home, I struggled with my identity. God took a hold of me and began His work within me. Not only did He transform me, but many of my friends who attended the University of North Texas with me.

It was being actively involved in various ministries on campus such as Steppers for Christ, Voices of Praise (VOP) Gospel Choir and Men of Virtue and Excellence, that I saw a community grow in grace and knowledge of the Lord. God had blessed us with a variety of artistic expressions. As my freshman year came to a close, VOP hosted the annual Gospel Fest.

It was at the conclusion of this event that my mother spoke these words to me: *The demands of ministry on your life will require you to be physically fit.* I must admit, those words didn't really connect much with me then, but the more I have grown in the ministry and seen the demands of it, I remembered those words. So, what began as a personal desire to develop my body has turned into a way to glorify God with my fitness.

A few years back when I began my fitness journey, I wrestled with how I could glorify God with it. I realized there were multiple benefits to becoming more fit, however my ultimate desire was to glorify Father. I wanted to be completely sold out for Him in this aspect of my life. As a result, I decided to create clothing gear that could represent the faith while people worked out. So in April 2015, I publicly announced *Wake Pray Train,* based off the foundational scripture 1 Timothy 4:7-8.

But have nothing to do with irreverent folklore and silly myths. On the other hand, discipline yourself for the purpose of godliness [keeping yourself spiritually fit]. For physical training is of some value, but godliness (spiritual training) is of value in everything and in every way, since it holds promise for the present life and for the life to come. (Amplified version)

We have since seen people from literally around the world representing their faith with our athletic gear. From Texas to Hawaii, to Afghanistan and Africa, God has blessed our movement and we are eternally grateful.

It is my desire that as you read this book, you will not only be filled with excitement and encouragement, but also have a longing to glorify God in your fitness as a Fit Christian.

PART I

The Warm Up

1

This chapter has been repurposed for this book, originally published in Conversations: Developing An Intimate Dialogue With God (Westbow Press, 2014).

Prayer is the vehicle by which we communicate with God. It is a silent or spoken conversation that we have with the Father. When communication takes place, it's about giving and receiving information, so prayer is all about conversation.

Whether planned or spontaneous, formal or informal, prayer should be offered sincerely to God through faith. Prayer is the believer's ACTS (Adoration, Confession, Thanksgiving, Supplication) directed to the Father and, in return, listening to His response.

You may wonder, "How does God speak to us?"

God speaks to us through many avenues: impressions of the

heart, with His audible voice (although this rarely happens), through one of His yielded vessels (e.g., preachers or believers), or via Scriptures.

Most times God initiates the conversation by speaking to us through the pages of His Word, but it's up to us to respond via prayer. It's when we respond through prayer that we complete this communication cycle.

The word *prayer* throughout Scripture seems to be exclusive to humans. The Bible speaks of other created beings being able to communicate with God (e.g., Job 1:6–7; Rev. 5:8–14) but it never classifies these instances as prayer. Maybe there's an element of helplessness caused by our inferiority or being marred by sin that creates the need to communicate with God, and request His help in matters. Whatever the case may be, prayer is the most powerful tool we have on Earth.

Prayer, as seen in Scriptures, can be viewed as the following:

- Communion with God (Phil. 4:4–7)
- Coming to God with praises and petitions (Eph. 1:15–23)
- Talking and listening to God (1 Sam. 3:2–14)
- Conscious dependence on God (2 Cor. 1:9–11)
- Acknowledgement of our need for God (1 Sam. 1:9–17)
- Calling on God to intervene in our lives (2 Sam. 15:31)
- One way God makes His will known to us (Col. 1:9)

– Claiming God's promises and relying on His mercy, grace, and provision (Dan. 9:17–19)

Biblical History of Prayer

The Bible first mentions prayer in the book of Genesis. We see at the beginning of Scripture the Earth being populated. Then, after Abel's death, Adam and Eve bear another son, Seth, who was seen as the provision from God. Seth's son Enosh began to call on the name of the Lord or worship and communicate with God. Thereafter, worship of Yahweh (the Hebrew name of God) advanced and the word *pray* used in Gen. 18:3 and *prayer* used in 2 Sam. 7:27.

Throughout Scripture, we see various reasons that sparked men to pray. One of the melting pots of prayers offered to God is found in Psalms. In Psalm 6, we see prayer in the time of distress. In Psalm 9, we see the prayer of thanksgiving to God. Psalm 13 is a prayer of one in sorrow, whereas Psalm 19 is a praise of God's glory. Psalm 54 contains a confident prayer in a time of distress, while in Psalm 62, prayer is an affirmation of trust in God. Then Psalm 63 displays the need and longing for God.

Types of Prayer

Throughout the years, believers have remembered the types of prayer through a mnemonic that describes each one:

ACTS. As mentioned previously, this stands for Adoration, Confession, Thanksgiving and Supplication.

Adoration

If someone always came to you with a request but never gave thanks for what you did for him or her, how would you feel? The first type of prayer, in accordance with the progression by which we enter into conversation with God, begins with giving adoration or praise to the Father.

Scripture is filled with prayers of praise and prayers that begin with praise before a request is made. In Psalm 150, the psalmist declares, "Praise Him for His mighty acts and excellent greatness." In John 17, we see Jesus praying for His disciples. Then in Matthew 6: 9-13, Jesus gives us the model of prayer, known by many as the Lord's Prayer. In this prayer Jesus begins by giving adoration: "hallowed be thy name" or "holy is your name."

As you can see, praise is verbally giving adoration to God's greatness, goodwill, and grace. The Bible is filled with prayers of adoration, or praise to God.

A Few Points about Adoration

1. Adoration should be offered from the soul with your entire heart (Ps. 9:1; 103:1; 111:1; 138:1).
2. Adoration should be expressed verbally (Ps. 51:15; 63:3;

119:7; 171).

3. Adoration is given joyfully (Ps. 63:5; 98:4).

4. Adoration is offered continuously (Ps. 35:28; 71:6).

5. Adoration is admitting because God deserves our praise (Ps. 33:1; 147:1).

Biblical Examples of Adoration

* Hannah (1 Sam. 2:1–10)
* David (Ps. 119:164)
* Anna (Luke 2:36–38)
* Paul and Silas (Acts 16:25)

Confession

As we survey God's character, we see that He is forgiving. Although He has forgiven us of our past, present, and future sins, unconfessed sin can disrupt our sweet intimacy with the Lord. That's why we confess our sins privately and sometimes publicly when applicable (e.g., some illness that appears to be caused by unconfessed sins [James 5: 16]). Because God is holy, we should approach Him boldly yet with reverence and vulnerability.

A Few Points about Confession

1. It should be done humbly (Isaiah 64: 5–6).
2. The Bible encourages it (James 5: 16; Josh. 7: 19).

3. We should let go of the confessed sin and not cling to it (Prov. 28: 13).

Biblical Examples of Confession

* David (Psalm 51)
* Nehemiah (Neh. 1: 6–7)
* Peter (Luke 5: 8)

Thanksgiving

Along with adoration, giving thanks is imperative. Paul writes, "Give thanks in all circumstances; for this is the will of God in Christ Jesus for you" (1 Thess. 5: 18). Just as our Father loves to answer our prayers (sometimes in ways we don't want), He also loves to hear the words thank you.

A Few Points about Thanksgiving

1. It's God's will (1 Thess. 5:18).
2. It should be offered before meals (Acts 27:35).
3. It should be included in our prayers (Phil. 4:6; Col. 4:2).
4. It should be offered to the Godhead (Father, Son, and Spirit) (Ps. 50:14; 1 Tim. 1:12).

Biblical Examples of Thanksgiving

* David (1 Chron. 29:10–13)
* Jesus (Matthew 11:25–26)

* Paul (Col. 1:3–11)
* Angels and saints: Revelation 7:11–12

Supplications

Having a conversation with God can be seen as we give adoration, confess sins, give thanks, and ask for things for ourselves or others. The prayer of supplication is asking God for something, and this is usually seen in Scripture as petitions or requests.

Inquiry prayers are when we ask God for information. When these types of prayers are offered to God in Scripture, it's to request an answer concerning personal distress or discomfort. In Joshua 7:6–9, an inquiry prayer was offered when Joshua was stunned by defeat. We see him keeping with the ancient ritual of mourning by tearing his clothes, putting dust on his head and falling before God's presence until evening. In Isaiah 45:11, an inquiry supplication was offered to God because of problems understanding God's Word.

A lesson I've learned through Scripture and personal experience is that God doesn't rebuke our sincere questions when our faith experience challenges Him. And God isn't obligated to always give us the answer we desire when we desire it.

Petitions, which are similar to inquiries, are prayers calling on God to act on our behalf concerning something. An investigation of petitions throughout Scripture displays requests by men and women. Remember that not asking means not receiving (James 4:2).

Lastly, we see prayers of supplications in the form of intercessions. How often has someone asked you to pray for him or her? When a believer offer petitions for God to act on behalf of someone else, this is called intercession. According to Scripture, we aren't only encouraged to offer prayers on behalf of others (1 John 5:16), we're also commanded to do this (1 Tim. 2:1).

This type of prayer is also common in the Psalms as shown in the examples given earlier. Intercessions were seen in times of famine (2 Sam. 2:1) and discomfort (Job 7:11-21). Scripture also shows countless people we should intercede for: children (1 Sam. 1:27), friends (Job 42:7-8), the sick (James 5:14), our enemies (Matt. 5:44), those in authority (1 Tim. 2:1-2), and (by ministers) for parishioners (Phil. 1:4).

A point I want to reiterate about inquiries, as with other types of prayers, God doesn't rebuke our sincere questions when our faith experience challenges. However, it may be in these moments when Jesus' prayer echoes in the distance: "I am praying for them. I am not praying for the world but for those whom you have given me, for they are yours" (John 17:9–13).

A Few Things for Which We Can Pray

1. The Spread of the Gospel (Col. 4:3; 2 Thess 3:1)
2. Deliverance from Satan and evil men (2 Thess. 3:2)
3. Wisdom, strength, comprehension, and encouragement (Eph 3:14-16, 18-19)
4. Knowledge of God's will with all spiritual understanding (Col. 1:9)
5. Physical and spiritual healing (James 5:13-16)
6. Those in authority (1 Tim. 2:1-2)
7. Pray about all things in every situation (1Thess 5:16-18)

A Few Biblical Examples of Supplications

* Abraham – Genesis 18:23-32 (Intercession)
* Lot – Genesis 19:18-21 (Petitions)
* Job – Job 7:11-21 (Inquiry)
* Daniel 9:3-19 (Intercession)
* Thief On Cross – Luke 23:39-43 (Supplication)
* Jesus – Luke 22:32 (Intercession)

Strategic Prayer

When facing anything in life, having a strategy seems most effective in accomplishing things. Since being strategic proves to be valuable, here are five ways we can be strategic as it pertains to prayer.

• Be **Spontaneous**

Spontaneity in prayer requires a willingness to abandon your own agenda and adopt God's agenda. It means being flexible and surrendering to whatever He permits no matter what comes your way.

- Be **Specific**

We should feel confident as we approach the throne of grace boldly to obtain grace and find help in our time of need (Heb. 4:16). Because of such access, we can be direct and specific with God (Matt. 6:7).

- **Summon** The Right Way

When we approach God and ask Him for something, it implies that we have a need that we want to be met.

Ask yourself:

1. Is my request fair and helpful to everyone concerned?
2. Is my request in line with the Word of God?
3. Will it draw me and/or others closer to God?
4. What is my part in answering this prayer?

- **Supplicate** with all your heart

  ◦ Pray aloud

  ◦ Write down distractions

  ◦ Keep a prayer journal

- Never **Stop** Praying (1 Thess. 5:17)

Praying without ceasing doesn't mean to break our communication, but rather having a persistence or regularity in our conversation to the Father. This is summed up perfectly in *The Minister's Personal Handbook.*

In all honesty, the vast majority of us waste minute after minute every hour in useless daydreaming and wandering thoughts – wasting precious time that could be spent in prayer. If we would learn to captivate these minutes in prayer, we would discover what it is to walk and live in prayer. (p.263-264).

The image below is a picture of my hand and it serves as a strategic way to pray. It is a guide for those I pray for. It is something I've seen for years and have adopted into my personal prayer time. I am not sure the originator of this, but it has been a blessing in aiding me in whom to pray for, by simply using each finger as my prayer guide.

Thumb: Pray for those closest to your heart such as family and friends.

Index/Pointer Finger: Pray for those that point you to truth such as your pastor, mentors, and ministers.

Middle Finger: Pray for the leaders of the church, locally and globally. Also, pray for leaders of government.

Ring Finger: Pray for those in trouble, persecuted and/or in pain.

Pinky Finger: Pray for those unnoticed, abused, orphaned and deprived.

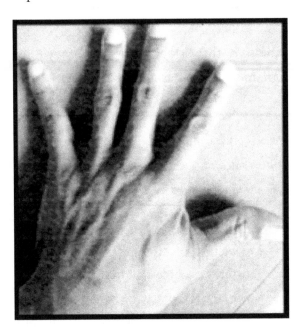

Key Benefits of Prayer

Prayer is vital to the growth of the believer. It pumps up our faith in God's faithfulness (Acts 27: 21-26) and produces boldness for Christ by purifying our motives for ministry service (Acts 4: 23-24, 29-31). The common thought among believers is that "prayer changes things," however prayer doesn't always change circumstances. If we surrender to God's will, prayer can change our perspective to trust God's providence. When believers fail to pray it results in that believer's loss, because nothing can replace the joy of communing with the Father. It should be our first response instead of our last resort (Acts 12: 1-5).

Therefore, as believers, we should devote ourselves to prayer (Col. 4: 2), by humbly seeking the face of God with all our heart (2 Chron. 7: 14-15) and asking according to His will (1 John 5: 14-15) with fervor both regularly and persistently (1 Thess 5:17; Acts 2: 42; James 5: 16).

Prayer and Fasting

"Fasting helps express, deepen, confirm the resolution that we are ready to sacrifice anything, even ourselves to attain what we seek for the kingdom of God." – Andrew Murray

So He said to them, "This kind can come out by nothing but prayer and fasting." (Mark 9:29)

Many people believe that fasting is good for the purpose of purifying the body, while others see it beneficial for physical and/or cosmetic reasons. However, Scripture teaches a great deal about fasting, and yet none is for these practical reasons. Also, the scriptures seem to only command fasting as it pertained to the children of Israel observing the Day of Atonement (Lev. 16:29; 23:27), which was a national fast that included adults to children.

Along with the above benefits, fasting also has its potential dangers such as trying to manipulate God. We see this in Isaiah 58:1-5, whereby the people seem to show an outward eager to hear from God, but they were quarreling and having poor relationships with others. They were going through the motions thinking God would see them, not realizing God saw their motives and exploitation.

Fasting can also be potentially dangerous when people attempt to impress others by doing so. I often see people who are fasting post about it on social media or tell others what they are doing, when Jesus clearly states in Matthew 6:16-18 the proper way to fast. A person can become legalistic in thinking this is the way to please God or be approved by God, without understanding that the only way to please God is by faith. For without faith, it is impossible to please Him (Hebrew 11:6).

Application

I once heard a story given by Dr. Brian English, who is a good friend of mine. He described himself as having nomophobia. I must admit when he first mentioned the condition, I thought it was something he made up. However, nomophobia is the irrational fear of being without your mobile phone, such as being without battery life or signal. He goes on to describe his "no mo phone Brian" occurring in situations when an individual experiences anxiety by not having access to their phone.

He continues to talk about how this fear caused him, like many others, including myself, to have chargers in multiple places so that no matter where we are, we always have a power source. All we have to do is plug in, so that we can have great power. But in our spiritual walk, we also have a great power source that we can plug into regularly. Just like we keep our phones plugged in all day to avoid drainage, we have access to the Father through prayer to always be charged 100%.

Remember that prayer is not some mystical thing that only the elite engage in. It is simply a conversation that we have with the Father. As with all dialogue, it is about giving and receiving information. So as you enter into a regular conversation with the Lord, remember also that fasting can be a vital part of that relationship. Fasting allows more time for us to enter into conversation with Him because it clears our hearts to be more attentive and confirms our seriousness to hear from the Lord.

It is my prayer that this brief study of prayer jumpstarts your lifelong communication with the Father, allowing you to experience the joy that comes with communing with Him and always trending towards 100% power.

2

Introduction to Spiritual Disciplines

This section is a combination of spiritual and physical training. For the next 31 days you will enjoy a daily spiritual protein and workout of the day (WOD).

Introduction to Spiritual Disciplines

In 1 Timothy 4:7, Paul exhorts Timothy to "exercise yourself toward godliness." This is translated in a few other passages as "train yourself for godliness (ESV), "train yourself to be godly" (NIV) or "discipline yourself for the purpose of godliness" (NASB). Timothy is basically encouraged to train his soul just as an athlete trains his body. So in essence, spiritual disciplines are about developing habits of holiness and guarding ourselves from the dangers of laziness and heartless obedience. The reason this is valuable is found in verse 8, "godliness is profitable for all things" because "it holds promise for the present life and also for the life to come" (ESV).

Spiritual disciplines are the practical ways we obey the command of 1 Tim. 4:7. The goal of every spiritual discipline is godliness. Godliness is another way of describing holiness, sanctification and Christlikeness. Essentially, the purpose of spiritual disciplines is intimacy with Christ and conformity both internally and externally to His character. Spiritual disciplines are exercises or activities that one engages in habitually to bring them closer to God and thus becoming godlier in character and behavior.

Dallas Willard categorizes these as Disciplines of Abstinence (1 Pet 2:11) and Disciplines of Engagement (Mark 2:11). For a detailed look at this, grab a copy of his book *The Spirit of the Disciplines*. Here is a quick look at 10 of them:

1) Prayer – in which one spends time talking to God (Dan. 6:10; Col. 4:2)
2) Meditation – in which one contemplates on God's word, or other things worthy of such attention (Ps. 1:1-2; Ph. 4:8).
3) Fasting – usually accompanied with prayer, in which one abstains from food (Neh. 1:4; Acts. 13:2-3; 14:23)
4) Singing – through which one can praise God and be edified (Ps. 71:23; Acts16:25)
5) Giving – by which we can please God and be blessed (Heb 13:16; Acts 20:35)
6) Assembling – where we can exhort one another Ps. 122:1;

Heb 10:24-25)

7) Hospitality – showing kindness to strangers, which often results in a blessing (Heb 13:2)

8) Teaching – which usually benefits the teacher more than the student (Heb. 5:12-14)

9) Service – where we see God's compassion and love flowing through us to those in need. (Col. 3:22-24; Matt. 20:25-28)

10) Bible Reading – allowing the words of God to strengthen and encourage our faith (2 Tim. 3:16-17)

Such spiritual activities help to discipline or train us to be godlier. So as you begin your FIT – Faithful In Training – journey, it is my desire that you train the total man: spirit, soul, and body.

3

Creating S.M.A.R.T. Goals

Michael Hyatt once said, "goals poorly formulated are goals easily forgotten." We usually utter goals like, "exercise more often" develop a closer walk with God" and we don't realize why these types of goals fail often. An excellent book to read about goal setting is Michael Hyatt's *Your Best Year Ever*. But here is a high-level checklist about S.M.A.R.T. goals.

Specific

Does the goal clearly define expectations in terms of actions and outcomes?
Does the goal avoid oversimplification or generalities and use action words instead?

Measurable

Is the goal results based?

Does the goal define specific metrics (quality, quantity, etc.) that can be objectively measured?

Achievable

Is the goal challenging but within reason?

Do I have skills and experiences necessary to achieve this goal, or do I know the right people to assist?

Is the achievement of my control or another's?

Relevant

Does the goal clearly connect with my true motivation?

Is God glorified with the accomplishment of this goal?

Time-bound

Does the goal specify a date or amount of time needed for when each goal needs to be completed?

Source: Latham, Gary P., and Edwin A. Locke, "Enhancing the Benefits and Overcoming the Pitfalls of Goal Setting" Organizational Dynamics (2006) *slightly rephrased*

With any goal, you have to be diligent and not lazy about achieving them. Here is a comparison chart showing the difference between the diligent and the lazy.

Proverbs	The Diligent	The Lazy
10:4	Becomes rich	Becomes poor
10:5	Gathers early and considered wise	Sleep during harvest and causes shame
12:11	Will be satisfied	Follows frivolity
12:24	Will rule	Will be alienated/forced labor
20:13	Love to awake and have food to eat	Love sleep and remain poor
21:5	Careful plans lead to an abundance	Make hasty plans
28:19	Reap abundance through hard work	Weeds grow slowly and eventually overbearing.

PART II

Wake Pray
T.R.A.I.N.

Temple Transformation
Refocused Mindset
Aspiring Health
Inspired Lifestyle
Normalized Discipline

4

Day 1 - Race Yourself

Are you concerned about others? Are you trying to beat someone else? DO you focus on the "competition" more than yourself? So often in life, we are worried about the competition instead of being concerned with being the best version of self-possible. My parents always told me, "nobody can do what you do, like you do it" so today instead of worrying about others, direct that energy in making yourself better.

Daily Prayer: *"Father, because we oftentimes ask for what we already have, today teach us what to pray for. Amen"*

Spiritual Discipline Focus: Prayer
Write Your Own Prayer Today

Workout Of The Day (WOD):
300 – Gideon Workout
100 Pull Ups
100 Push Ups
100 Squats

Record Your Time:

5

Day 2 - Be About It

"In all labor there is profit, but idle chatter leads only to poverty" – Proverbs 14:23

Have you ever heard the adage, "don't talk about it, be about it." Oftentimes, we talk about all these amazing goals we will accomplish. We speak about the what-ifs, however, we should start seeing things as "why not?" Why not me? Why not today? Why not start today instead of putting it off for tomorrow? In the above passage, Solomon encourages us that if we want to see a profit, we can't merely talk about it, we must be about it. Work diligently. Work consistently. In due time we will reap a harvest if we faint not.

Daily Prayer: *"Father, open our eyes to the opportunities you give us to develop fruit in our lives. Amen"*

Spiritual Discipline Focus: Prayer
Discover a prayer partner and commit to praying throughout this month's journey.

WOD:
High Intensity Interval Training (HIIT)
Hiit Session: Treadmill/Elliptical/Bike/Jump Rope

Beginner

- 5 minute warm up

- 10 rounds of 20 seconds sprinting and 40 seconds rest

- 5 minutes cool down

Intermediate

- 5 minute warm up

- 10 rounds of 30 seconds sprinting and 30 seconds rest

- 5 minutes cool down

Advance

- 5 minute warm up

- 10 rounds of 40 seconds sprinting and 20 seconds rest

- 5 minutes cool down

6

Day 3 - Be Diligent

The plans of the diligent lead surely to plenty, but those of everyone who is hasty surely to poverty. – Proverbs 21:5

We live in a world of instant gratification. We have drive-thru restaurants and even created the fast-casual restaurants (e.g. Chipotle). We want everything fast, and will even pay extra just for convenience. Think about it, a 20oz Dr. Pepper cost more than a 2 liter bottle. Even when it comes to fitness goals, we are under the impression that what took years to create, can be corrected within days.

There are legitimate ways to jumpstart your fitness in a short period of time, like a 24 day challenge from Advocare (shameless plug http://robertadvocare.com). However, you cannot correct everything overnight that took years to create. There are many plans, pills and physical trainers selling you on the idea that you get the gains or losses you desire quickly. But, be mindful of this scripture, meditate on it: *the plans of the diligent lead surely to plenty, but those of everyone who is hasty surely to poverty.*

So often we contrast diligence with laziness, but in this passage, diligence is opposed, not to laziness, but moving quickly. The individual who manages his affairs without consideration or trying to gain quickly leads to empty. Albert Barnes commentary states, "Undue hurry is as fatal to success as undue procrastination." Often we think we are going to get the immediate results we desire, and when we don't see them, we often give up. So my encouragement is for you is to change your perspective. See your fitness journey as a lifestyle change and it will take time, but celebrate the small wins along the way.

Daily Prayer: *"Father, may our goal be to love and make you famous, not acquiring riches. Amen"*

Spiritual Discipline Focus: Prayer
Pray for a stranger: Ask God to place you in position today to pray for someone you haven't prayed for before.

WOD: Tabata (20 seconds hard 10 seconds rest and repeat 7 times)
Push Ups
Squats
Jumping Jacks
Upright Rows with desired weight

Record Your Time:

7

Day 4 - Space Yourself

Remember sometimes you need to space yourself from the grind. Constantly fighting your giants, opposition, or self can be taxing and you need time to rest and recuperate. Take a few moments each day for quiet time; time to realign yourself with purpose and refuel your passion. Also, be sure to allow your body time to rest and recover; it is through rest we can see optimal gains.

Daily Prayer: *"Lord, you are my strength and you shield me from all evil. Amen"*

Spiritual Discipline Focus: Prayer
Read The Disciple's Prayer (Matt 6:9:15)

WOD: Today's workout involves rest, reflection and restating our goals.

What is your why? What is the pain you are experiencing that brings about a desire to change? What is your true motivation?

8

Day 5 - 2 >1

Two are better than one, because they have a good return for their labor: – Ecclesiastes 4:9

Accountability is vital. We see this in all aspects of life. Why is two better than one? Because they have a good return for their labor.

In a spiritual sense, accountability can be helpful in the battle to overcome a specific sin. An accountability partner (AP) can be there to encourage you, rebuke you, teach you, rejoice with you, and weep with you. An AP also helps see the blind spots in your life. Like a quarterback, we are waging war against the opposition, and oftentimes we fail to see the edge rusher coming from our blind side. However, the accountability partner can assist as a guard against those attacks.

Also, sometimes the small drips in our lives, when gone undetected, can eventually create floods. So why should we have accountability partners as it pertains to glorifying God with our fitness? Our AP can also be helpful in the battle to overcome weight loss or muscle gain. They can be there to encourage you, teach you, rejoice with you, spot you, and weep with you. They should also be driven to seeing the same goals in their life. When we approach our physical fitness alone, we will still see the results, however like the Scripture states, we can have a better return for on our labor when we fight together with someone.

Daily Prayer: *"Father, grant your servants an increasing desire to do your will together. Amen"*

Spiritual Discipline Focus: Prayer
Host a prayer phone conference
Record the names of those who joined you

WOD: "Boxed In"
4 Rounds of 20 Box Jumps and ¼ Mile run

9

Day 6 - First Step Is Taking A Step

*Do not despise these small beginnings, for the Lord rejoices to see the work begin...*Zechariah 4:10

Sometimes the goal before you is so large, you feel overwhelmed and don't know where to start. However, the only way to climb a mountain is to take one step at a time. Your goal before you might seem like a mountain, but you have to get started.

Create a daily productivity schedule and remember that God rejoices when the work begin. Although the above passage is talking about the work of the Lord, you can be sure that if God is telling us not to despise small beginnings when it comes to His work, why do we despise the small beginnings when it comes to natural things as well. Take each day, one day at a time, and over the course of days, weeks and months you will see the accumulation of something great.

Daily Prayer: *"Father, give me a single mind to trust you completely. Amen"*

Spiritual Discipline Focus: Prayer
Pray for each person who joined your prayer conference call.

WOD:
Box Jump 10 sets 10-1 Reps (No Rest)
Pull Up 10 sets 10-1 Reps
Decline Pushup 10 Sets 10-1 Reps (No Rest)
Weighted Carry (Dumbbell/Kettlebell) 10 Sets Run 25 yards (Rest 30 seconds)

Rest as directed between exercises, where 0 seconds for rest, only rest as long as it takes to set up the next exercise. When you see 10-1, you will perform 10 reps the 1st set, nine the 2nd, eight the 3rd, and so on.

10

Day 7 - Discipline Determines Destiny

You cannot possess what you won't pursue – Robert L. Wagner

There are dreams and goals that many of us desire. We have thought about it, we have written them down, and we have even created vision boards. However, unless you make the effort to pursue that thing, you will not possess it. Only runners obtain the prize. Only fighters win the match. If you don't attempt the shot you are guaranteed a 0% chance to make it.

Martin Luther King, Jr. once said, "if you cannot fly; run, if you cannot run; walk, if you cannot walk; then crawl. By all means keep moving." It will take work, it may cause pain, but as Anthony Robbins said, "there are two kinds of pains in life: the pain of discipline and the pain of regret."

Discipline determines destiny! So if you want to possess it, by all means pursue it and make every effort to exercise discipline along the way, because the worst thing than the pain of discipline is the pain of regret.

What are you pursuing? What do you want to possess? How can someone coach, motivate or run with you?

Daily Prayer: *"Father, may we yield to the work of the Spirit at work in and through us. Amen"*

Spiritual Discipline Focus: Prayer
Devote to praying daily

WOD: "Park Workout"
Explosive Pushup 3 Sets 5 Reps
Parallel Bar Leg Raise 3 Sets 10 Reps (Optional: Lying Leg Raise)
Sprinter Step Up on Bench 3 Sets 10 Reps
Pullup with 10 Second Hold 3 Sets 4 Reps
Bulgarian Split Squat 3 Sets 10 Reps (Each Leg)
Finish with 20-30 Second Sprints 10 Sets

11

Day 8 - Brace Yourself

We can't get to where we think we are already – Robert L. Wagner

On the road to success we have to assess where we are. Significant progress toward that goal is made when we lay aside unnecessary weight, which could be seen in the false reality that we are where we hope to be or the lack of belief that we can get there. It is when you start believing not when others believe that you start making movement toward your goals. So therefore brace yourself as you assess, analyze and advance. Brace yourself for the naysayers along the way, and brace yourself from yourself. Instead of listening to your inner voice of defeat, tell yourself, "Today I will overcome."

Daily Prayer: *"Father, may the power of your love rule over what we or anyone says or does. Amen"*

Spiritual Discipline Focus: Bible Reading
Read the book of Philemon
Record your greatest takeaway

WOD:
Dip 4-5 Sets 10-12 Reps (No Rest)
Burpee 4-5 Sets 10 Reps (No Rest)
Aligator Walk 4-5 Sets 10-12 Reps (No Rest)
Walking Lunge 4-5 Sets 10-12 Reps (Each Leg) (No Rest)

Record Your Time:

12

Day 9 - Value Thyself

We relish news of our heroes, forgetting that we are extraordinary to somebody too. – Helen Hayes

So often we tend to focus on the victories of those "giants" in our path, not realizing that we are giants in our own right. Growing up, my mother and father affirmed me often which led me to walk with a great deal of confidence and sought to excel in whatever I did. Yet there are times in my life when I minimized what I knew as something "common" knowledge.

There were times along this book journey, where this has played a part in its delay. Oddly enough, what is often common to us is extraordinary to someone else. We may not be experts to everybody, but to the right person we are. My encouragement is that today you learn to walk confidently in your own skin. Don't minimize what you know or what you can offer to someone else, because what is trash to one person can be treasure to another. Be Great!!!!

What have you procrastinated in presenting? What do you have to offer that you think is common, but gold to the right person? What resource can you give that may impact one?

Daily Prayer: *"Father, teach us how to manage our time, resources, relationships and lives better." Amen*

Spiritual Discipline Focus: Bible Reading
Read the book of Jude

WOD:
Set for a timer for 15 minutes
Do 15 Burpees 1st Minute
15 Crunches 2nd minute
15 Jumping Lunges (Rest Remainder of 3rd Minute)
Repeat 5x

13

Day 10 - Let's Talk About Lemons

Sometimes we are so quick to take what we have been given only to apply it the way we always have. We have all heard the saying, "take your lemons and make lemonade." However, those who are wise know to take the lemons they have been given, survey their needs and apply them appropriately. Applying them appropriately could mean making lemonade to refresh you or it could be using the lemons as a cleaning agent. There are so many benefits to using lemons, but if we stop short of seeking wisdom, we will miss out on the wonderful ways to use something sour for something special. Be Wise. Be Intentional!

Daily Prayer: *"Father, you don't have to remove the mountains before us,* however, *grant us wisdom to know if we should climb or walk around them. Amen"*

Spiritual Discipline Focus: Bible Reading
Read 1st Chapter of James

WOD:
Warm Up 5 minute on cardio machine of choice
Low Back Machine 1×12
Leg Extension 1×12
Leg Curl 1×12
Row Machine 1×12
Pec Deck 1×12
Lateral Raise 1×12
Bicep Curl 1×12
Triceps Machine 1×12
Ab Machine 1×12
15 Min. Jog

14

Day 11 - Ace Yourself

So often we see the lives of others and desire to be just like them. But, I want to encourage you that you were created to be you, and nobody can do you like you. You possess a greatness of gifts, talents and tons of creative wealth that if you don't unleash it, you will rob the next generation. It's okay to take ingredients from others, but always be unapologetically you. So today, take the first step to "Ace Yourself" because we are waiting on you, to give your offering to the world, so that we all can be blessed.

Daily Prayer: *"Lord, grant us favor to meet the right people with the right resources at the right time. Amen"*

Spiritual Discipline Focus: Bible Reading
Read Joshua 1: 1-9

WOD:
DB Flat Bench Press 3-4 Sets of 6-10 Reps
Leg Press 3 sets of 8-10 reps
Barbell Rows 3 sets of 8-10 reps
Leg Curls 3 sets of 8-10 reps
Barbell Bicep Curls 3 sets of 8-10 reps
DB Overhead Extension 3 sets 10-12 reps
Resting 60-90 seconds after each set

15

Day 12 - Spring Forward

Setting goals for ourselves can start off exciting and easily become a daunting task. The year has begun and I am sure many of us are thinking in the words of Paul "not that I have already obtained it" (Phil. 3:12a). We have goals of physical fitness, financial peace, promotion, etc.

I am convinced that if a person wants to receive the prize of an accomplished goal, they must first have proper awareness of what they are and what they are not. Many have started this year off with key goals in mind, but have stalled, abandoned or are nowhere close to achieving them. However, in order to reach the goal it requires maximum effort. Saul continues in his letter saying, "but I press on so that I may lay hold of..." thus an individual will not reach the goal until they first realize the need to improve and then it takes a springing forth.

Many of us have faced our giants and moved beyond the obstacle that face us, but we have become stagnant in thinking that we have arrived. We have yet reached the goal by which we set out to obtain. We must spring forward and focus our attention on that which lies ahead. We must…"forget what lies behind and reach (spring) forward to what lies ahead." Springing forward, or reaching forward, translates as stretching a muscle to its limitations to reach a goal.

One of my favorite movies is Rocky 4" and Tony "Duke" Evers said it best, *"no pain no gain."* In other words, until you take your body through rigorous pain you will not see the gains you desire to see; therefore we must push ourselves to the limit to reach the goals, dreams and aspirations we have set for ourselves. So as you set your annual goals, I hope that you use this as a reminder to Spring Forward in your pursuit of the ultimate prize.

What are some things that hinder you from reaching your goals? What will you take away from this excerpt? Have you made much progress this year? Where do you see yourself in the next 9 months?

Daily Prayer: *"Father, help us to press towards the higher calling and not focus on the things of this world. Amen"*

Spiritual Discipline Focus: Bible Reading
Read 1st Samuel 17

WOD:
Overhead Lunge 12 Each Side
Sumo Squat 15 Reps
Superman 12 Reps
Glute Bridge 12 Reps
Repeat 3x

Record Your Time:

16

Day 13 - Small Things, Big Value

When becoming more physically fit, we often tend to focus only on the big muscles; and while that's great, it's not until we give attention to the smaller muscles, that we start seeing real body transformation.

This is also true in our lives when we focus on just the big things, and fail to remember or see the smaller areas. King Solomon throughout Song of Solomon once echoed this thought as it relates to relationships by saying: *catch for us the little foxes...that destroy the vineyard.* Because in relationships, it's oftentimes those minor things that if left unattended, build up over time into something bigger, leading to major conflict. Remember that the small behaviors are the ones that aid and/or assist in the accomplishment of larger goals.

What is your biggest takeaway? What are 2 or 3 behaviors you're hoping to focus on and improve? What do you need assistance with?

Daily Prayer: *"Father, help us to identify the drips from the faucets in our lives that become deluges or a superabundant stream. Amen"*

Spiritual Discipline Focus: Bible Reading
Read Psalm 1

WOD: Stretch Day

17

Day 14 - Free To Fail

Failure is the salt that seasons success – Stan Toler

Did you know that many times success in life is a result of failed attempts? Did you know that Bill Gates watched his first business fall apart? George Steinbrenner bankrupted his basketball team before owning the Yankees. Or that Steve Jobs was booted from his own company before coming back and taking it to new heights? Don't be afraid to fail; if you want to be free to fail you have to overcome fears. Fear of being criticized, judged or seen as inadequate. My dad always said that "fear was simply false evidence appearing real." Therefore shake your fears off, and strive toward greatness. Don't rob future generation of the greatness or wealth inside of you. We are awaiting your greatness to be unleashed.

What is your biggest takeaway? What greatness are you waiting to achieve?

Daily Prayer: *"Father, thank you that these light and momentary afflictions that are preparing us for an eternal weight of your glory. Amen"*

Spiritual Discipline Focus: Bible Reading
Read Psalm 139

WOD: Shoulders
DB Military Press 4×12
Lateral Raise 5×12
Cable Upright 4×12
DB Front Raise 4×12
Shoulder Shrugs 4×12

Record Your Time:

18

Day 15 - Prayer

God, you are amazingly perfect and far more appealing than anything this world has to offer, you're so holy. I can't wait for your return. However, until then keep me focused on you to not fall into the cares of this world. I also ask for your daily provision. Father, I have blown it so many times, and I am grateful for your forgiveness. May my life be a reflection of your honor, glory, and grace to the world around me. You are eternal, unchanging God and I bless your name. Amen!

Spiritual Discipline Focus: Service
Display A.R.K. (Act of Redeemed Kindness) to a member of your church

WOD: Back

Wide Lat Pulldowns 5×10

Superset:

Close Grip T-bar rows 4×10

Wide Seated Rows – 4×10

Superset:

Bent over Barbell Rows 4×10

Straight Arm Cable Pulldown 4×10

19

Day 16 - Fix Your Eyes

A lady came to her spiritual advisor with a list of complaints about people in her organization. Her spiritual advisor filled a cup with water and asked her to do him the favor of walking around the building three times, making sure she didn't spill a drop of water. After having done so, he asked what she had noticed. She replied, "I didn't notice anything, since I was focused on making sure no water spilled from the cup I was carrying." He replied, "That's the point. If you will turn your focus on the main goal and follow after it, you won't have time to notice all the things you're complaining about."

So often we are consumed with the things that's going wrong, that we take our eyes off the prize. Wherever you want to end up, is where you should focus your attention.

Life is too short to focus on the negative things, let's turn our eyes to the things that matter most. Make today great!

Daily Prayer: *"Father, we commit our plans to you and submit to your rearrangements. Amen"*

Spiritual Discipline Focus: Service
Volunteer to clean your church one weekend this month

WOD: Chest
DB Incline Press 4×10
DB Bench Press 4×10
Superset:
Cable Flyes – 4×10
Close Grip Flat DB Press 4×10
Pushups 4 Sets Failure

20

Day 17 - Game Plan Your Success

Every year comes and goes, and for many of us, there are things we often leave on the table. It unfortunately becomes a year of regrets.

Sometimes we need to slow down and think through our decisions and devise a game plan while being flexible enough to know that we may need to re-strategize mid game. Whether this is applicable personally, professionally, relationally, socially, spiritually or financially we have left some "money" on the table. Many times this is due to our own efforts, but other times, it's because people make moves that we cannot control, and for whatever reason, we didn't have enough foresight to consider that. My encouragement is that you take some time to strategize and consider the different ways to play, while making the best use of the skills/talents in your hand.

Like you, I have been hit with disappointments, failures, successes, and everything else in my life. Yet, in all things I maintained a long-term perspective and made the necessary adjustments along the way. My desire for you/us is that this year will be the year "We Came, We Saw, and We Conquered."

Daily Prayer: *Father, may we live passionately on purpose. Amen*

Spiritual Discipline Focus: Service
Leave a letter of hope on someone's car window

WOD: Legs
Barbell Squats 4×10
Leg Press 4×20 (10 wide and 10 close)
Leg Extensions 4×10
Straight Leg Deadlifts 4×10
Lunges 4×10

21

Day 18 - Embrace Yourself

It is very difficult for us to look into the mirror and not instantly identify our blemishes. Likewise, when we give our offering to the world, while others are blessed and think highly of our presentation, many times we identify the flaws in it. We seek perfection and not progression. Today, I want you to "embrace yourself." Although, we all have room to improve, you are not always as great as others say and surely not as bad as you think.

Lastly, as you are racing and bracing yourself, you will encounter bumps and bruises along the way. Whether they are the words of naysayers or days when life happens, I want to encourage you to "embrace yourself." Love yourself!

I love this reflection from Paul found in Romans 8:28 which says, "and we know that all things work together for the good…" Although all things that happen to us are not good thing, they can all work out for our good. Embrace yourself!

Daily Prayer: *"Father, thank you for the comfort that is given in the midst of trials. Amen"*

Spiritual Discipline Focus: Service
Ask a single parent if you could serve them (i.e. wash dishes, read kids a bedtime story, mow their lawn, etc.)

WOD:
DB Swing
Single Leg Squat
DB Row
Superman Pushup
Jump Rope
Repeat 5x

Do each exercise for 30 seconds and rest 30 seconds

22

Day 19 - No Quick Fixes

He who works his land will have abundant food, but he who chases fantasies lacks judgment. (Proverbs 12:11)

Have you ever seen an Instagram photo of someone that made you drop your jaw? This could be in the form of fitness competitors, celebrities, magazines, etc. So often the image that is marketed to us, creates unrealistic expectations for ourselves. We wish, hope and even begin to chase the fantasies that are displayed before us and never work our farms, or as the adage goes we desire the grass that is greener on the other side only to find out it is artificial turf. We often forget about what we have been given, and only focus on what we don't have.

This is evident in marriages when a spouse chases fantasies, rather than spending time tending to his/her own family. We see this with finances, fitness, or even our gifts and talents. Maybe this is why in the parable of the talents, the individual with the 1 talent went and buried his portion because he didn't have two or five talents (Matt. 25:14-30). Diligent work results in plenty of food, but when we chase after things mentally, physically, etc. the work doesn't get done and thus it produces lack in our lives. When we forget the work that is before us and chase after other things, it shows our lack of judgment. So often these people we admire, have personal chefs, unlimited resources, take 1000 pictures until the right one is produced and still edit it, or even take shortcuts to get the results they desire (like steroids, plastic surgery, etc).

International teacher, speaker, evangelist and advisor, Myles Munroe, once said, *your success is not determined by what you have, but by what you do with what you have.* So grind on!

Daily Prayer *"Father, give us this day our daily allotment. Amen"*

Spiritual Discipline: Service
Send a care package to a college student with an encouraging note.

WOD: Hiit Session: Treadmill/Elliptical/Bike/Jump Rope-
• 5 minute warm up

- 10 rounds of 20 seconds sprinting and 40 seconds rest
- 5 minutes cool down

Beginning 20/40 split, Intermediate 30/30 split, and Advance 40/20 split

Day 20 - The Source Provides Resources

The proper use of resources maxims potential and the abuse of resources destroys potential. – Myles Munroe

God is our source. God uses various things as resources to assist us in accomplishing our purpose and goals. However, when we don't properly understand the purpose of our resources, it can potentially thwart our progress. The unleashing of your potential is tied directly to your ability to understand and obey their properties. It is not until we understand our resources, and how to operate them from within, that we are able to see maximum gains.

God grants unto us resources so that we can accomplish the purpose of our existence here. When you walk into a gym, your gym membership affords you certain resources, however when you are clueless to those resources they can cause great harm. So often I see people in the gym, using equipment that is designed for one thing, but they are not obeying the laws that govern that resource.

Here are a few recommendations:

1) It's okay not to have full understanding. However, what are you going to do with the lack of knowledge.

2) It's up to you to discover and develop your understanding of the resources you have access to.

3) If you don't know the purpose of that resource, ask questions. Find a professional, or even seek online tools that can aid you in properly using the resource.

4) Determine now to use all that has been granted to you.

5) Don't allow fear to hinder you.

Daily Prayer *"Father, grant unto us the wisdom to succeed. Amen"*

Spiritual Discipline: Service
Ask a group of friends to pick up trash surrounding your church's neighborhood.

WOD:

Upright Row 8 Sets 3 Reps
Rack Pull 4 Sets 10 Reps
Incline DB Press 4 Sets 10 Reps
Six-way Shoulder Raise 3 Sets 10 Reps

24

Day 21 - Make Better Decisions

You won't leave where you are until you decide it's not where you want to be – Robert L. Wagner

There is great power in decision. Someone once said: *what mind can conceive, man can achieve.* Our decisions affect every area of our lives. The direction of where we are going has been driven by the decisions we make each day. Therefore, making better decisions leads to better living. Today I encourage you to make better decisions and experience better results. Small or large, trivial or transformative, strong decision making helps cultivate our lives for the better and shape our culture, whether good or bad.

Daily Prayer: *"Father, may we become decisive in our pursuit of progress. Amen"*

Spiritual Discipline: Service
Deliver cookies or love gift to local first responders.

WOD: Stretch Day

25

Day 22 - Pace Yourself

We have talked a lot about your goals, success and overall life potential. My encouragement in this reflection, is that in all things, pace yourself. Ecclesiastes 9:11 says, "the race is not given to the swift, nor the battle to the strong...*but to him who endures to the end.*" (Italics Added) It may have taken the snail or turtle some time to get to the ark, but they eventually made it. So pace yourself, give yourself room to grow and never compare yourself to others. You are exactly where you should be in life, just strive to go a little farther each day.

Daily Prayer: *"Father, may we maintain an eternal perspective. Amen"*

Spiritual Discipline: Silence/Solitude

Today begin to incorporate silence in your prayer time. Spend 2 mins. in solitude after speaking to God.

WOD:
Front Squats6 Sets x 10/8/6/6/6/3
Leg Press 3 Sets 10 Reps
Walking Lunges 2 Sets 10-15 Reps
Superset:
Leg Extension 2 Sets 20 Reps
Leg Curls 2 Sets 20 Reps

26

Day 23 - Prepare For Tomorrow

Our conscious and subconscious goals have tremendous power to motivate us. Our perceived goals are statements of faith about the future. – Edward R. Dayton

We are where we are today because of the many choices we made on yesterday/yesteryear. Are you satisfied with where you are? Have you thought about where you want to be? Are you making the necessary choices to ensure a better tomorrow?

As we quickly approach the final stretch of the book, I want to ask, have you made progress towards the goals you've set? If not, what choices are you making today that will ensure tomorrow's success?

Daily Prayer: *"Father, thank you for leading me daily. Amen"*

Spiritual Discipline: Silence/Solitude
Spend 4 min solitude after speaking to God.

WOD:
Incline DB Press 6 Sets 10/8/6/6/6/3
Chest Dips 3 Sets Failure
Cable Triceps Extension 3 Sets 10 Reps
Cable Crunches 4 Sets 15 Reps

27

Day 24 - Accountability

Accountability enables others to identify the blind spots in our lives
– Robert L. Wagner

I am a fitness competitor. One of my goals was to compete in the Ronnie Coleman Classic (bodybuilding competition) and I accomplished it! I went on to compete in a few more and placed 2nd in one and 2nd in another. However, I knew I hadn't reached my potential. I knew I could be leaner, eat cleaner and be overall meaner. I wanted to achieve my best self and I knew I could. So I hired a trainer/coach.

The one thing I loved about the process was that I had more accountability. I checked in weekly with pictures and updates and he adjusted my plan as needed. He has, in essence, become my accountability partner (AP). Accountability enables others to identify the blind spots in our lives.

Someone once said, *"everyone has blind spots and everyone needs help to see problem areas that we tend to overlook or minimize."*

My encouragement for you is to identify someone that can hold you accountable for accomplishing your goals (i.e. monthly, career, fitness, development, etc.). Achieve more! Cut out the distractions! Be even more diligent!

What is your biggest takeaway? Who have you identified as an "AP"?

Daily Prayer: *"Lord, thank you for those in my life who are able to walk alongside in purpose. Amen"*

Spiritual Discipline: Silence/Solitude
Spend 6 min solitude after speaking to God.

WOD: 2 Mile Walk/Jog

28

Day 25 - Disagreements Don't Detour

A few years ago, I attended training on how to handle conflict. Disagreements are inevitable when you have two or more people together. We all come from different walks of life, see things differently, and ultimately just have different viewpoints. . But, disagreements aren't the issue, it's how we handle those disagreements that matters.

We must keep in perspective that one, we are a part of the same team, and two, we are pursuing the same mission. So often when we disagree, we lose sight of these two points.

Shaq and Kobe didn't see eye to eye much in the early 2000s, but when the whistle blew, they understood they were on the same team—the Lakers— and fighting for the same mission—the championship. Because they understood that, they went on to four championships in five years and won three in a row.

Even though we don't see things alike, we can still accomplish great things when we lace up our sneaks, hear the whistle blow and remember we are on the same team fighting for the same mission.

Daily Prayer *"May we never lose sight of our common goal. Amen"*

Spiritual Discipline: Silence/Solitude
Spend 8 min solitude after speaking to God.

WOD:
Deadlift 6 Sets 10/8/6/6/6/3
Hyperextension 3 Sets 8 Reps
DB Leg Curl 3 Sets 6 Reps
Seated Calf Raise 3 Sets 15 Reps

29

Day 26 - Don't Wait For Permission to Be Great

Have you ever seen someone with an incredible amount of potential and yet they sit on it? Or you've seen someone with something of value to offer, but yet they keep it to themselves? So often we live our lives waiting for a symbolic *knight* ceremony before we act according to our greatness. Don't slow down for others to recognize your greatness, live it and let them catch up to you.

Daily Prayer *"Father, may our greatness be unleashed for Your glory. Amen"*

Spiritual Discipline: Silence/Solitude
Spend 10 min solitude after speaking to God.

WOD:
Front Lat Pulldown 6 Sets 10/8/6/6/6/3
Underhand Lat Pulldown 3 Sets 8 Reps
Upright Row 3 Sets 10 Reps
Incline DB Curl 3 Sets 10 Reps

30

Day 27 - Seek Progression

Stop beating yourself up because it's not perfection, but rather rejoice for the progression – Robert L. Wagner

Too often we get caught in the perfection syndrome. However, seek progression in your work; you'll be amazed one day at how far you have grown and how you can bless your generation along the way.

Daily Prayer *"Father, thank you that I haven't already attained it, but pressing towards the mark is my daily delight. Amen"*

Spiritual Discipline: Silence/Solitude
Spend 12 min solitude after speaking to God.

WOD: Rest

31

Day 28 - Be Obedient

Your obedience might not produce immediate happiness, but when you realize what He protected you from as a result, you will be ecstatic.

In what way has God's protection been seen in your obedience?

Daily Prayer *"Father, thank you for your protection. I am grateful that you love me and lead me. Amen"*

Spiritual Discipline: Solitude & Journaling
Spend 10 min solitude after speaking to God and then journal

How is God dealing with you? What do you hear Him say? Where are you being led?

WOD:

Ab Crunch 4 Sets 25 Reps

Leg Curls 5 Sets 10 Reps

Straight Leg Deadlifts 4 Sets 10 Reps

Chest Press 4 Sets 10 Reps

Pec Deck Flyes 4 Sets 10 Reps

Standing Bicep Curls 4 Sets 10 Reps

32

Day 29 - Growth By Suffering

One of the greatest detriments to the Church's growth and ability to thrive around Emperor Constantine era (306 to 337 AD) was the absence of persecution.

According to Luke 21:11-12, God will grant the church opportunity to bear witness in the midst of persecution. "*God uses the persecution and suffering of his people to spread the truth of Christ and to bless the world.*" (John Piper). Instead of hiding, sulking, complaining or fighting, use the season of suffering as an opportunity to proclaim God's faithfulness.

Daily Prayer "*Father, your hands of comfort and strength have watched over me and held me in the night.*"

Spiritual Discipline: Solitude & Journaling
Spend 10 min solitude after speaking to God and then journal

When faced with suffering how do you respond? What are some actions you can take to change this? How often do you stop and think about the consequences or positive outcomes of your actions?

WOD:
Lat Pulldown 4 Sets 10 Reps
Seated Rows 4 Sets 10 Reps
Shoulder Press 4 Sets 10 Reps
Lateral Raises 4 Sets 10 Reps
Triceps Pressdowns 4 Sets 10 Reps
Overhead DB Triceps Extension 4 Sets 10 Reps
Russian Twists 100 Reps (50 Each Side)
Hanging Leg Raise 20/19/18/17/16/15/14/13/12/11/10 (5 second rest between each rep count)
Plank 90 Seconds
Crunches 2 Minutes non-stop

33

Day 30 - God Provides

For most of my life, I had a speech impediment. I would stutter often especially at the beginning of a sentence. You have no idea how that can intimidate a young person in front of people. Yet, God graced me with a personality to be almost fearless in those moments.

Oddly, when I would stand before people to proclaim His faithfulness, my stuttering stopped and my speech rate slowed. My biggest takeaway wasn't anything super spiritual, although I believe God wanted me to accurately communicate biblical truth. What I learned is how to breathe before speaking and how to organize my thoughts. Even though sometimes I have to rearrange a sentence, I am still fearless to proclaim.

I am who I am today by the grace and love of Father exercised through practical means. I encourage you to reflect on His grace in your life, extract the practical ways He has provided and developed you, and encourage others to do the same.

Daily Prayer: *"Father, I give you my imperfections and let your grace be sufficient. Amen"*

Spiritual Discipline: Solitude & Journaling
Spend 10 min solitude after speaking to God and then journal

Which imperfection you have that need to be submitted to Christ? How does your faith provide a foundation for the work you do? What imperfection do you need to overcome?

WOD:
Weighted Crunches 4 Set 25 Reps
Seated Calf Raises 4 Sets 15 Reps
Leg Press 5 Sets 10 Reps
Leg Curls 5 Sets 10 Reps
Wide Chest Press 4 Sets 10 Reps
DB Curls 5 Sets 10 Reps
Preacher Curls 5 Sets 10 Reps

34

Day 31 - Breaking Through

I first read this poem as a seminarian reading a book on Hermeneutics, which is the art and science of biblical interpretation. I have ironically used this for a lot of things in my life. So often we give up too soon not realizing our breakthrough could be just an inch away. Keep pushing!!!!!

"Peering into the mists of gray
That shroud the surface of the bay,
Nothing I see except a veil
Of fog surrounding every sail.
Then suddenly against a cape
A Vast and silent form takes shape,
A great ship lies against the shore
Where nothing has appeared before.

Who sees a truth must often gaze
Into a fog for many days;
It may seem very sure to him
Nothing is there but mist-clouds dim.
Then, suddenly, his eyes will see
A shape where nothing used to be.
Discoveries are missed each day
By men who turn too soon away."

Clarence Edward Flynn

Daily Prayer *"Father, we actively wait on you. Amen"*

Spiritual Discipline: Solitude & Journaling
Spend 10 min solitude after speaking to God and then journal

Do you have a difficult time waiting? Do you sometimes get agitated when your needs are not in your time? In what ways does God develop patience in you?

WOD:
Hack Squats 4 Sets 10 Reps
Romanian Deadlifts 4 Sets 10 Reps
T-Bar Rows 6 Sets 10 Reps
Rear Delt Flyes 5 Sets 10 Reps

Machine Shoulder Press 5 Sets 10 Reps
Single Arm Triceps Pressdowns 5 Sets 10 Reps

PART III

F.I.T. Christians

F.I.T. Christians
(Faithful In Training)

35

Daily Protein Bites

Daily Proverbial Protein Bites

Listed below are 90 daily protein bites. These can be posted online, written somewhere, or quoted for the next 90 days to motivate you to greatness. If you do post online, be sure to use #WakePrayTrain #ProteinBites

1. Just because you are not in the same place as others doesn't mean you are not exactly where you should be.

2. In order to reach your goal maximum effort is required.

3. If you only attempt what can be done, how will you ever discover what can't.

4. Become the person they regret walking away from.

5. All men fall, but it's the great ones that get back in the fight.

6. Don't allow the failures of yesterday to affect your today.

7. Use your setbacks to propel you forward.

8. Be careful of the tunnels you walk in, because the light at the end might be an oncoming train.

9. Turn your lack into seed for your harvest.

10. Don't gripe about what you grant.

11. When others try to speak to their storms to cease, choose to speak to the One who controls all things.

12. Instead of reminding yourself of your problems, remind yourself of God's promises.

13. If it doesn't open, stop trying to make it your door.

14. Pursuit takes excellence, endurance and integrity.

15. When you think you can't, accomplish will soon follow.

16. Movement towards your goals happen when you begin believing not when others believe for you.

17. Significant progress is made when we lay aside unnecessary weight.

18. Highly progressive people are often separated not by talent but by belief.

19. You can't get to where you think you already are.

20. Progress towards our goals begin when we are clear of where we currently are.

21. Be mindful of the applause of others. Cheers for the underdog are soon transferred to another.

22. What is successful isn't always effective.

23. What we don't prioritized gets minimized.

24. Being successful to prove haters wrong is focusing on the wrong person to please.

25. Obstacles and opposition offer us an opportunity to honor Father.

26. Don't make someone a priority that treats you as a convenience.

27. God's favor is exponentially greater than our failures.

28. What God starts He completes.

29. Trials have a way of bringing us to Our Father's feet.

30. Don't miss your opportunity worried about your opposition.

31. What doesn't kill you doesn't always make you stronger, it could be the very thing that disables you.

32. Listen not to give a quick response but listen to fully understand.

33. Awake from your dreams to accomplish much work.

34. That which seems impossible, only takes small steps in the right direction to see incredible progress.

35. Guide your mouth with your heart and prepare your heart with the Word of God (Prv 16:23).

36. The words you speak should be gracious and timely. This means knowing a word is sometimes not needed, just your presence.

37. Don't allow people to redefine loving you in a way that accommodates their wants.

38. You won't leave where you are until you decide it's not where you want to be.

39. The challenge is not in failing but in taking the continual risk without losing excitement to try again.

40. We cannot expect to be challenged in our comfortability.

41. Every closed eye is not sleeping and every open eye is not seeing.

42. Don't judge an entire life upon one season.

43. Don't fail to see the good in others and the bad in self.

44. If you keep hooking a certain type of fish, maybe you should change your bait.

45. When thoughts arise contrary to God's way, wise people rehearse, refresh and reiterate the Word.

46. All godly people in Scripture are people of prayer.

47. God took a man with no woman and brought forth Eve, then took a woman with no man and brought forth Jesus. Give your lack to God!

48. Surround yourself with key people that can positively affect your flame.

49. Stop focusing on your problems and start focusing on the problem solver.

50. In order to accomplish your goals, you must have great focus.

51. God is so creative He can put a window where there is no wall just to bless you.

52. Our patience can be seen in our trust in the Lord's timing.

53. What happens to us isn't always good, but it always works out for our good.

54. Prayer presupposes a belief in the personality of God.

55. God's grace is as old as His existence and as current as our present need.

56. Some don't need encouragement in the form of an earful, but rather an empty ear fully formed and ready to be there and listen.

57. Stop beating yourself up because it's not perfection, but rather rejoice for the progression.

58. Be the person you always dreamed you would be.

59. Don't be discouraged by small beginnings; it may have taken the snail weeks or months to get to the Ark, but it finally did.

60. Plans in life change often due to unforeseen circumstances, but if you aren't flexible you will break.

61. Be stubborn with where you want to go, but be flexible with how you will get there.

62. Oftentimes the cost of missing out on the opportunity could prove costlier than messing up in the opportunity.

63. Choose to be successful by making successful choices daily

64. Jesus is the answer not the alternate.

65. Some things don't need resuscitation, they need resurrection.

66. God has not forgot!

67. If you only attempt what can be done, how will you ever discover what can't.

68. Sometimes procrastination becomes procrastinever; act now!

69. The external problems in relationships are rarely the real issue. Get to the root of the issue and not the fruit of it.

70. Every artist began as an amateur; therefore, wherever you are in your development be encouraged and continue to develop.

71. Patience brings about the revelation of deceit.

72. The only way to adequately steer a ship is when it's moving forward.

73. Prayer is conversation and conversation is a dialogue, not merely a monologue.

74. Man wants to enjoy "God's presents", but God wants man to enjoy "His presence".

75. Courage is doing what you're afraid to do.

76. Courage is the mastering of our fears not the absence of them.

77. Focus on the people and not the resources.

78. Instead of being quick to give an opinion, be slow to offer up prayer.

79. The plan of God doesn't stop because of domestic or foreign adversaries.

80. Everyone falls, but will you get up.

81. A key to success is finding life in your failure.

82. Pain in your current yields future gains.

83. Be so loving and kind that the blind can see.

84. First give yourself to God, then everything you have can be freely given.

85. Don't wait to prepare; prepare as you wait.

86. It's okay to outgrow circumstances and/or people.

87. Forgiveness is like going to the edge of a cliff and throwing a Frisbee as far as you can, knowing you will never see it again.

88. There are nutrients in manure, therefore find the blessing in your mess.

89. Don't waste time counting sheep to cure insomnia, talk to the Shepherd.

90. Pray focusing on the one who controls all things and not focusing on your circumstances.

36

Rise. Slay. Eat. (Nutrition)

So, whether you eat or drink, or whatever you do, do all to the glory of God. 1 Cor. 10:31

It is important for us to slow down in such a hurried world. So often we eat with distractions and lack of focus. It's important to occasionally slow down so you can shift your relationship with your food into a healthier direction and decision.

As we look into nutrition, I want you to consider taking time each day and actually experience eating. We have been given teeth and taste buds for a reason, so that we can find satiation with our food.

As a small exercise, I would like for you to take one small piece of a food you enjoy and look at the color, the texture and notice its shape. Think about how it came to be and praise God for His creativity and thank Him for His provision. Take a deep breath and enjoy what God has granted. After you do this, ask yourself: *What did it taste like? What did you think once you actually concentrated on eating it?*

Being healthy requires dedication. When things are in motion like they are in our lives, it requires more energy to pump the brakes and prepare us. The words my father uttered to me more than 20 years ago still rings true today, "proper preparation prevents poor performance." We can't expect to perform well if we are not prepared. We can't think that we will crush our goals when we are ill-prepared. So here are a few tips I have adopted from a few sources.

1) Attack Your Preparation Ahead Of Schedule

Have you ever thought about how a masterpiece at a restaurant can be accomplished so quickly by a chef? They have what are called prep cooks. When you are doing something that doesn't require your undivided attention, use it to make preparation for the big day; chop your veggies, wash your fruit, cut your fruits, etc. By preparing these ingredients ahead of time, can shave some serious time when you are ready to make all meals.

2) Tackle Your Cooking In One Day

I normally cook my meals for the week on Sunday afternoon. I turn the grill on, throw on the meat, and make all the sides, before packaging it all up. Don't make it a stressful event, have a meal prep party!

3) Reward Meals

I know you have heard of cheat meals before, but I honestly hate the term. Cheat meals have the connotation that you're cheating on yourself, so, I like to use the phrase "Reward Meal," Reward yourself for a job well done, reward yourself for a successful week, and reward yourself so that you can continue along the journey. However, ensure you are having a reward meal and not reward day.

4) Outsource it!

One of the things I have done in the past has been to outsource my preparation. Whether it is the entire preparation, or just the hard part of thinking about what I needed to eat, you can consult with an experienced dietician or trainer to get yourself free of that menial task.

5) Prioritize your label review

I know that looking at nutrition labels can be overwhelming, but honestly, you only need to focus on a few nutrition facts: protein, carbs and fat (the three essential macros) and sugars and sodium. I've trained myself to look quickly at these nutrients and it's saved me a tremendous amount of meal prep and eating time.

6) Healthier Fast Food Choices

I know sometimes we can't help it, but when you find yourself at a fast food restaurant, always choose the healthier choices.

7) Protein On Deck

There will be times when you're caught off guard; however, always having a protein shake on hand can be very beneficial.

Basics of Nutrition

This information is not intended to diagnose, treat, cure or give advice on treating illnesses. Always be sure to consult with your physician before beginning new plans. With that being said, this section is intended to wet your appetite and give a brief overview of nutrition.

What are Macros?
There are four macronutrients macros that you will find on a USDA nutritional facts label: Fat, Carbohydrates, Protein and Alcohol. Each of these play an important role within the body, and therefore need to be carefully weighed as we spend time providing energy or fuel to our bodies. These are the four places you get your calorie intake from.

What is a calorie?

A calorie is, in essence, a unit of energy. It is a measurement. Carbs and Protein both contain the same amount of energy – 4 calories per gram, and fat contains 9 calories per gram. In addition, alcohol provides 7 calories per gram. So always be mindful of your intake.

Carbohydrates

There are two types of carbs: Simple (sugars) and Complex (starch and cellulose). Carbs are not really considered essential for daily survival. However, without them you are not able to perform optimally in a few areas. Without carbs your muscle recovery time diminishes, your exercise performance can decline, and you can also lose mental focus. Carbs also play a part in your metabolic rate.

Protein

Protein is an often feared word among people who don't want to look like "those" guys. But protein is vital for muscle development and fat loss. Protein aids in the formation of enzymes and neurotransmitters, which help to regulate a multitude of body processes. Protein feeds our muscles, and without it, consequently, our muscles can deteriorate.

Fat

While it makes sense to lose fat, we must not deny ourselves of it. Fat is necessary for our survival. It aids in normal development and growth, and hormone production and balance. The three main types of fat are saturated, unsaturated and trans. Trans fat are to be stayed away from at all cost, because they increase your risk of things like heart disease, cancer, and obesity.

Saturated fats can also be linked to heart disease when consumed in excess. Saturated fats should be replaced by unsaturated (monounsaturated and polyunsaturated). Unsaturated fat is the best fat to consume and is found in coconut oils, nuts, avocado, fish and olive oil. This help reduce cardiovascular issues and can improve overall brain function and blood cholesterol.

37

Diets vs. Lifestyle Change

We live in a fast food society. We want everything yesterday, and when we are not experiencing the quick results we think we should see, oftentimes we quit altogether. Personally, I do not like the term diet because it seems like we are killing something: killing my vibe, killing my fun, killing the taste of good food. However, eating should be enjoyable and as someone said, *"eat to live and not live to eat."* Most people also associate diets with quick fixes, which is why I would much rather a person replace the verbiage of diet with lifestyle change.

So why don't they work?

Some would argue that diets don't work across the board because they are restrictive and hard to stick to long-term. By seeking the latest trends in diets it encourages yo-yo dieting by jumping from one fad to the next. They can also interfere with metabolism. Since many people are seeking extreme weight loss in an extreme time frame, they seek after extreme dieting. These are often associated with eating too few calories. Without enough energy, the body begins to conserve calories which can lead to a host of undesirable side effects including mood swings, fatigue, loss of focus, lower immune system, and reduced muscle tissue resulting from the body breaking it down to create energy.

It all comes down to calories: if you want to gain weight you must consume more calories than you expend (calorie surplus). If you want to lose weight you must get a caloric deficit. For example, to lose 1lb a week, cut 500 calories a day = 3,500 calories/week, therefore an awareness of calories is important if you are trying to lose weight. When being mindful of calories, one must also pay close attention to portion sizes. Many restaurants give too much to eat and the best way to offset this is eating homemade meals. This way you can control and monitor what you are taking in.

Another method to monitoring calorie intake is by keeping a food diary or journal. By tracking your consumption you are better prepared to make necessary adjustments as needed. Ask yourself: What changes can be made? Where can calories be eliminated? Are my meals balanced? Do I have healthy eating habits?

HEALTHY EATING BEHAVIORS

When developing healthy eating behaviors you are planning and preparing well. As another person once said, "*those who fail to plan, plan to fail*" so plan well. Planning well includes setting goals, creating a meal plan, writing a shopping list, and either cooking in bulk or cooking the night before. Ultimately you have to change your attitude towards food and your goals, maintain a positive focus and have realistic expectations if you are going to be successful in eating more healthy.

38

6 Basics For Food Prep

1) Food Containers with Lids

- The best way to portion control or monitor what you are eating is by storing your food in airtight containers each day.

2) Plastic Bags

- This is valuable when it comes to separating snacks, proteins, fruit, or other food products.

3) Poultry Scissors

- This is essential as it pertains to cutting your proteins and trimming your fat. You can purchase your food trimmed already, however you can save a lot of money by doing it yourself. Also, cooking your food with the fat can add to the overall flavor and moisture.

4) Grill

- Propane Grills, Electric Grills, and/or Smokers are valuable resources with meal prep. This allows you to cook large quantities of food in an easy and less time-consuming manner.

5) Food Scale

- It is a must-have. In order to calculate macronutrients (i.e. protein, carbs, fat, etc.) you need to measure your food. Measuring your food is also important as it pertains to making adjustments along the way. You cannot adjust what you are unaware of taking in.

6) Measuring Cups

- This is important to measure your fruit, greens, carbs, etc.

39

Fit Christians Master Food List

Looking and feeling good is a lifestyle, not a quick fix. It takes effort and hard work. It's an active process of becoming aware of the foods you consume and ultimately just making healthier choices. I have included a master list of food items for you to choose from.

Along with proper eating, you also want to make sure you are hydrating sufficiently. Water, not only boost immune systems and aids in increased energy, but it also helps move the toxins out of your system, that would otherwise they will be reabsorbed. So, make sure you drink at least 4 liters of water per day if you are male, and at least 3 liters of water if you are a female. Always consult with your doctor or nutritionist for best results.

MASTER FOOD LIST

This list should be used to make the best choices from each food category. You may substitute freely within each category any time you need a change of pace.

PROTEIN

Beef (4-6oz):	Dairy:	Poultry(4-6oz) :	Seafood (4-6oz):
Ground beef	Whole Eggs	Chicken breast	Tuna
(90% or leaner)	Egg whites	Ground	Salmon
Filet	Cottage Cheese	Chicken breast	Cod
Sirloin steak		Rotisserie Chicken	Tilapia
Flat iron steak		Turkey breast	Red Snapper
Round / flank		Ground turkey	Halibut
Beef Jerky		breast (90% lean)	Shrimp
			Crab

In a pinch for time?

Substitute:

Advocare Muscle Gain Protein

Advocare Meal Replacement Shakes

(http://robertadvocare.com)

Premier Protein – 30g Protein 5g Carbs

NON-STARCHY VEGETABLES

Asparagus	Cucumbers	Peppers
Cabbage	Green beans	Spinach
Carrots	Lettuce	Sprouts
Cauliflower	Mushrooms	Squash
Celery	Onions	Tomato

FRUITS

Apples	Cherries	Pears
Bananas	Grapefruit	Pineapple
Blueberries	Oranges	Plums
Cantaloupe	Peaches	Raspberries
		Strawberries

STARCHY CARBOHYDRATES

Beans	Quinoa	
Brown Rice	Red potatoes	Waffles/
Cream of rice	Sweet potatoes	Pancakes
Oatmeal	Wheat Bread	White Potatoes

FATS

Nut butter	Olive oil	Paul Newman's oil &
Peanut butter	Flaxseed oil	vinegar
Heavy whipping cream	Coconut oil	Nuts

"FREE FOODS"

Hot Sauce / Spices	Lime juice	Low Sodium
Cucumber	Mushrooms	Seasonings
Dry Seasonings	Mustard	Scallions
Garlic	Onions	Sugar-free gum
Lettuce	Pepper	Sugar-free Jell-O

FREE BEVERAGES

Water	Coffee (easy on sugar)	Sparkling water
Tea	Diet Sodas	Flavor additives

If you need to calculate your nutritional information you can use resources like

http://nutritiondata.self.com

My FitnessPal

40

Sample Meal Plans

I have included two sample meal plans for both male and female. Remember, you can track the macronutrients or calories via various food tracking apps. Feel free to modify these sample meal plans using the Fit Christians Master Food List.

Female Sample Meal Plan #1

Breakfast:
2 whole eggs and 3 Egg whites
1 packet of oatmeal (low sugar)

Snack:

1 apple

Protein shake (30g)…Premier protein drink or another type of protein from a vitamin shop

Lunch:

4oz Chicken breast
1 cup of Greens (broccoli, green beans, asparagus)

Snack

6-8oz of Greek Yogurt
1oz of Almonds

Dinner

4-6oz Protein (chicken, steak, turkey, etc.)
1 cup veggies

Late Snack

4-6oz Cottage Cheese / 4-6oz Greek Yogurt / Protein shake

Female Sample #2

Breakfast:
3-4 Egg whites
1 packet of oatmeal (low sugar)

Snack:

2 String Mozzarella Cheese

1oz Mixed Nuts

Lunch:

4-5oz Chicken breast

1 cup of Greens (broccoli, green beans, asparagus)

½ cup of Brown Rice, ½ sweet potato or Baked potato

Snack

4-5oz of Greek Yogurt

1oz of Almonds

Dinner

4-6oz Protein (chicken, steak, turkey, etc.)

1 cup veggies

½ cup of brown rice or ½ sweet potato, etc.

Late Snack

4-6oz Cottage Cheese / 4-6oz Greek Yogurt / Protein shake

Pre Workout Snack

Branch Chain Amino Acids (BCAAs) and Protein Shake

Post Workout Snack

Meal Replacement Shake

Male Sample #1

Breakfast
3 Eggs
3 Egg Whites (EW)
1 Cup Oatmeal
1 Orange

1st Snack
8oz Fruit Greek Yogurt
1oz Nuts

Lunch
8oz Chicken
1 Cup Spinach
6oz Sweet Potatoes

2nd Snack
1 Medium Fruit
1oz Mixed Nuts
3 Sticks String Cheese

Dinner
8oz Chicken
1 Large Sweet Potato
2 Cups Salad
1 ½ tbsp. Reduced Fat Salad Dressing

3rd Snack
Protein Shake – 30g 5g (or less) Carbs

Male Sample #2

Meal 1:
1/2 cup oatmeal made with water
7 egg whites cooked with 1 yolk
1/2 cup strawberries

Or

1 cup whole-grain cereal
1 cup 1% milk
1 piece fruit
1 Tbsp. peanut butter

Snack
2 String Cheese w/ 1oz Mixed Nuts

Lunch
Large baked potato with skin (3-4″ in diameter)
1 cup green veggies
6oz. sliced turkey

Snack
Protein Shake (Premier or Boost)

Meal 5
6 oz. lean steak
6-8 stalks asparagus or 2 cups salad (very light dressing)

Late Snack

4-6oz Cottage Cheese / 4-6oz Greek Yogurt / Protein shake

Pre Workout Meal
8oz Chicken ½ Cup Asian Jasmine Rice

Post Workout Meal
6oz Chicken
1 cup Asian Jasmine Rice

41

8 Ways To Handle Disappointments

The interesting thing about life and fitness is that at some point or another, we all face disappointment. Disappointments as some say, "is a fact of life."

In my years of coaching, training, and varying leadership positions, I have learned that when we don't deal with disappointment it creates a road of discouragement, despair, and ultimately devastation. So, ask yourself, how do you handle disappointment? How do you deal with the pain that comes along with it? Whether it comes from personal or professional issues, what do you do to overcome it?

Here are 8-ways to quickly pick yourself back up after disappointment surfaces:

1) Use it as fuel

Frustrations can become wildfires and consume us, or it can be used as wood thrown into a controlled fire. One of the things I continually work on is not allowing frustration to consume me, but instead using it to fuel my passion and propel me into my destiny. Channel your frustration to attack your goals more vigorously and you'll begin to see progress.

2) Stay the course

When we allow disappointment to create a road of discouragement, despair and devastation we are veer off the desired course for our lives. My father always told me to H.A.L.T. before making decisions. So, I encourage you that whenever you are Hungry, Angry, Lonely, or Tired (H.A.L.T.), take a break before your decision takes you off course.

3) Remain Positive

One of the hardest things to do in dealing with disappointments is to remain positive; especially when you don't feel that you are being properly rewarded for your efforts. You have to remember that oftentimes people are watching and they are counting on you, so don't lead them astray. Even our momentary negativity can cause long-lasting negative results. Stay positive!

4) Realize it's their loss and someone else's gain

I have always had the thought that when people overlook me,

it's their loss and my gain. Have you ever had a relationship end and then the person of your dreams was discovered? Referencing back #1, the 1998 NFL Draft, Randy Moss passionately wanted to be drafted by the Dallas Cowboys, but when they decided to go in another direction, he used that frustration as fuel to make them regret that decision. That same season, the Dallas Cowboys lost in convincing fashion to Randy Moss and the Minnesota Vikings. The Cowboys then realized their loss and the Vikings realized their gain as Moss went on to become a legendary receiver.

5) Let it out (don't bottle it up)

Whenever you experience disappointment, one thing you must always remember is to not hold it within. You must let it out! One time I got horrific news about something I wanted. I felt I was qualified and on my way, but when the team went another direction, instead of lashing out, I remained professional, walked away, took a deep breath and reminded myself of who I was and where I was going. I had to remind myself at that moment, I am not the sum of this decision, and I will not bottle it inside. Find a productive outlet and let it out!

6) Get some perspective (Stepping stone or Stumbling block)

As I mentioned before, accountability partners (AP)mare those who are able to see the blind spots in your life. As you think about heroes, how many of them accomplish great things alone? (Batman had Alfred and Robin, and even Jesus had 12 disciples) When you are faced with disappointment, consult with your team and get some perspective on how you can use it as a stepping stone to success, rather than a stumbling block to destruction.

7) *Practice what you preach*

If you are who you say you are, regardless if people see it or not, be true to yourself. Don't shrink back! Remain true to your guiding principles. I used to say, "he who listens to himself is foolish, but he who talks to himself is wise." Sometimes "self" will tell you to give up, throw in the towel, or it's not worth it, but you have to tell "self" who you are and why you do what you do. Practice what you preach, even if no one else is there to listen.

8) *Remember God is Sovereign*

At the end of the day, we have to remember that "...all things work together for good." If we believe that God is truly sovereign, then we should also understand that nothing happens that God did not permit to take place. He knows all, sees all, and is involved in the overall process. Trust God's heart when you can't seem to figure out His way. He cares for you more than you will ever realize and always has your best interest in mind.

Remember that life is full of disappointments; however, it's up to you to properly respond to them in order to achieve greater success and avoid despair.

42

7 Tips For Success

The fitness journey can be a lonely journey sometimes. It rewards you with both highs and lows. In my time of training I have learned a few tips that I would love to share with you as it pertains to getting the most out of yourself and becoming a better you.

1. Get Your Mind Right

The first thing in anything you do is deciding that you are going to actually do it. You can't walk until you take the first step. You can't get fit until you first decide that you need to.

I have learned that it's not just what you want, but rather what you're desperate for. There are a lot of people that want to change, but not many who are desperate for a change. Many people declare that they want the Lord, but it's not until they grasp that: *as the deer pants for the water, so my soul longs after thee,* that they get the real motivation spark for growth.

2. REWARD Yourself

Each and every week I engage in a Reward Meal. Taking time out for simple rewards and pleasures can refresh you along the way. It provides the personal satisfaction of knowing that I have had a successful week, and it provides the vital ingredient of celebrating small victories.

3. RELAX, RELATE, RELEASE

There is tons of research about the benefits sleep has regarding overall performance. Without getting too technical, sleep has an amazing effect on recharging your brain for the next day. Our bodies go in and out of sleep cycles, which are about 90 minutes in length. During these sleep cycles, there is a delivery of protein to your muscles for repair and growth. So sleeping is very important and should be embraced and not avoided.

4. CHANGE IT UP

Our bodies are highly adaptable. In order to not hit plateaus, you have to be sure to change it up from time to time. I observe people sometimes when they enter the gym. And I see them using the same equipment and doing the very same routines. I can almost predict where they will go next. Now if I can do that, don't you think your body can also predict what you're about to do. God has equipped our bodies to be adaptable, so if you really want to see "change," take your body through a series of shocks, by changing up what you do and how you do it.

5. STRETCH It Out

The older I get the more important this has become in my life. Stretching helps to improve your overall flexibility and range of motion. Another good benefit is that stretching allows you to get your game face on. When you begin your stretching you realize that in a matter moments your work out will begin, and it prompts you to be motivated. Also, stretching is key in the reduction of soreness after workouts, so remember to stretch before and after.

6. CHALLENGE Yourself

The old adage, "no pain no gain" is so true. In everything

in life, we experience struggle before the growth. Toddlers experience the discomfort of teething, teens the discomfort before puberty; even the Bible speaks about the suffering that produces character in Romans 5:2-4. If you want to grow in your fitness journey you can't be afraid to experience a little discomfort. Get out of your comfort zone and attack your discomfort, and you'll be happy that you did.

7. REMEMBER YOUR "WHY"

Times will become difficult and sometimes you won't see the progress you want, but you have to remember why you began. Your why has to be greater than just trying to be "summertime fine." A lifestyle of health and wellness is not limited to just the summer, it is year round. My why is to simply Glorify God through my fitness and health. What's your why? Take time to discover it, and I guarantee it will help fuel you to where you want to go.

43

Sample Full Workouts

Male Sample Full Workout

WORKOUT 1: CHEST, TRICEPS, ABS (MULTI-JOINT)

EXERCISE
Bench Press 4 sets (10-12)
Incline Dumbbell Press 3 sets (10-12)
Decline Smith Machine Press 3 x (10-12)
Dips 3 x (failure)
Close-Grip Bench Press 4 sets (10-12)
Cable Crunch 3 x (failure)

WORKOUT 2: SHOULDERS, LEGS, CALVES (MULTI-JOINT)

EXERCISE

Barbell Shoulder Press 4 x 10-12

Alternating Dumbbell Shoulder Press (Standing) 3 x 10-12

Smith Machine One-Arm Upright Row 3 x 10-12

Squat 4 x 10-12

Deadlift 3 x 10-12

Walking Lunge 3 x 10-12

Standing Calf Raise 3 x 10-12

Seated Calf Raise 3 x 10-12

WORKOUT 3: BACK, TRAPS, BICEPS (MULTI-JOINT)

All exercises 3 sets 10-12 reps (unless otherwise noted)

EXERCISE

Barbell Bent Over Row 4 sets 10-12

Dumbbell Bent-Over Row

Seated Cable Row

Barbell Shrug 4 sets 10-12

Barbell Curl

Barbell or EZ-Bar Preacher Curl

Reverse-Grip Barbell Curl

Barbell Wrist Curl

WORKOUT 4: CHEST, TRICEPS, ABS (SINGLE JOINT)

All exercises 3 sets 12-15 reps

EXERCISE
Incline Dumbbell Fly
Dumbbell Fly
Cable Crossover
Triceps Pressdown
Overhead Dumbbell Extension
Cable Triceps Extension Crunch
Standing Oblique Cable Crunch

WORKOUT 5: SHOULDERS, LEGS, CALVES

EXERCISE
Dumbbell Lateral Raise 3 sets 12–15
Barbell Front Raise 3 sets 12–15
Dumbbell Bent-Over Lateral Raise 3 x 12–15
Leg Extension 4 x 12–15
Leg Curl 4 x 12–15
Seated Calf Raise 3 x 12–15
Leg Press Calf Raise 3 x 12–15

Female Sample Full Workout

WORKOUT 1: Legs Abs

Leg Press 3×15
Squats 3×12
Hack Squat Machine 3×15
Stiff Leg Deadifts 3×12

Leg Extensions 3×12
Variety of Ab Exercises 8×30

WORKOUT 2: BACK, DELTS, BICEPS, CALVES

Calf Raises 6×15
Pulldowns 3×12
One Arm Dumbbell Row 3×10
Seated Cable Row 3×12
Dumbbell Lateral Raise 3×10 each way (side and front)
Barbell Curl 3×12
Incline Dumbbell Curl 3×12

WORKOUT 3: CHEST, TRICEPS, ABS

Abs 5×25
Flat DB Press 3×15
Incline DB Press 3×15
Dumbbell Flyes 3×12
Tricep Pushdowns 3×12
Dips 3×12

WORKOUT 4: Legs (Glutes)

Romanian Deadlifts 3×15
Barbell Hip Thrust 3×10
Squat 3×12
Wide Leg Press 3×10
Leg Curl 3×10
Walking Lunges 3×20 (10 each leg)

WORKOUT 5: SHOULDER, BACK, ARMS

Shoulder Press 3×10
Wide Pulldown 3×12
Lateral Raise 3×12
Superset: Upright Row 3×10
Seated Cable Row 3×12
Cable Curl 3×12
Superset: Overhead Extension 3×12
Abs 8×30

44

Fitness Challenges

Follow each day's reading and exercise. Also, be sure to post your challenge completions online using hashtag and challenge name.

Corinthian Crunch Challenge

o Day 1: 1 Corinthians 1 & 20 Crunches

o Day 2: 1 Corinthians 2 & 25 Crunches

o Day 3: 1 Corinthians 3 & 30 Crunches

o Day 4: 1 Corinthians 4 & 35 Crunches

o Day 5: 1 Corinthians 5 & Rest

o Day 6: 1 Corinthians 6 & 40 Crunches

o Day 7: 1 Corinthians 7 & 45 Crunches

o Day 8: 1 Corinthians 8 & 50 Crunches

o Day 9: 1 Corinthians 9 & 55 Crunches

o Day 10: 1 Corinthians 10 & REST

o Day 11: 1 Corinthians 11 & 60 Crunches

o Day 12: 1 Corinthians 12 & 65 Crunches

o Day 13: 1 Corinthians 13 & 70 Crunches

o Day 14: 1 Corinthians 14 & 75 Crunches

o Day 15: 1 Corinthians 15 & 80 Crunches

o Day 16: 1 Corinthians 16 & 85 Crunches

o Day 17: 2 Corinthians 1 & 90 Crunches

o Day 18: 2 Corinthians 2 & 95 Crunches

o Day 19: 2 Corinthians 3 & 100 Crunches

o Day 20: 2 Corinthians 4 & REST

o Day 21: 2 Corinthians 5 & 105 Crunches

o Day 22: 2 Corinthians 6 & 110 Crunches

o Day 23: 2 Corinthians 7 & 115 Crunches

o Day 24: 2 Corinthians 8 & 120 Crunches

o Day 25: 2 Corinthians 9 & 125 Crunches

o Day 26: 2 Corinthians 10 & 130 Crunches

o Day 27: 2 Corinthians 11 &135 Crunches

o Day 28: 2 Corinthians 12 & 140 Crunches

o Day 29: 2 Corinthians 13 & 145 Crunches

o Day 30: Prayer and REST

Church Letter Challenge

o Day 1: 10 Squats & Galatians 1

o Day 2: 11 Squats & Galatians 2

o Day 3: 12 Squats & Galatians 3

o Day 4: 13 Squats & Galatians 4

o Day 5: 14 Squats & Galatians 5

o Day 6: 15 Squats & Galatians 6

o Day 7: 16 Squats & Ephesians 1

o Day 8: 17 Squats & Ephesians 2

o Day 9: 18 Squats & Ephesians 3

o Day 10: 19 Squats & Ephesians 4

o Day 11: 20 Squats & Ephesians 5

o Day 12: 21 Squats & Ephesians 6

o Day 13: 22 Squats & Philippians 1

o Day 14: 23 Squats & Philippians 2

o Day 15: 24 Squats & Philippians 3

o Day 16: 25 Squats & Philippians 4

o Day 17: REST DAY

o Day 18: 26 Squats & Colossians 1

o Day 19: 27 Squats & Colossians 2

o Day 20: 28 Squats & Colossians 3

o Day 21: 29 Squats & Colossians 4

o Day 22: 30 Squats & 1 Thessalonians 1

o Day 23: 31 Squats & 1 Thessalonians 2

o Day 24: 32 Squats & 1 Thessalonians 3

o Day 25: 33 Squats & 1 Thessalonians 4

o Day 26: 34 Squats & 1 Thessalonians 5

o Day 27: 35 Squats & 2 Thessalonians 1

o Day 28: 36 Squats & 2 Thessalonians 2

o Day 29: 37 Squats & 2 Thessalonians 3

o Day 30: Prayer and REST

Proverbs Pushup Challenge

o DAY 1: Proverbs 1 / 10 Reps

o DAY 2: Proverbs 2 / 11 Reps

o DAY 3: Proverbs 3 / 12 Reps

o DAY 4: Proverbs 4 / 13 Reps

o DAY 5: Proverbs 5 / 14 Reps

o DAY 6: Proverbs 6 / 15 Reps

o DAY 7: Proverbs 7 / 16 Reps

o DAY 8: Proverbs 8 / 17 Reps

o DAY 9: Proverbs 9 / 18 Reps

o DAY 10: Proverbs 10 / 19 Reps

o DAY 11: Proverbs 11 / 20 Reps

o DAY 12: Proverbs 12 / 21 Reps

o DAY 13: Proverbs 13 / 22 Reps

o DAY 14: Proverbs 14 / 23 Reps

o DAY 15: Proverbs 15 / 24 Reps

o DAY 16: Proverbs 16 / 25 Reps

o DAY 17: Proverbs 17 / 26 Reps

o DAY 18: Proverbs 18 / 27 Reps

o DAY 19: Proverbs 19 / 28 Reps

o DAY 20: Proverbs 20 / 29 Reps

o DAY 21: Proverbs 21 / 30 Reps

o DAY 22: Proverbs 22 / 31 Reps

o DAY 23: Proverbs 23 / 32 Reps

o DAY 24: Proverbs 24 / 33 Reps

o DAY 25: Proverbs 25 / 34 Reps

o DAY 26: Proverbs 26 / 35 Reps

o DAY 27: Proverbs 27 / 36 Reps

o DAY 28: Proverbs 28 / 37 Reps

o DAY 29: Proverbs 29 / 38 Reps

o DAY 30: Proverbs 30 / 39 Reps

o DAY 31: Proverbs 31 / 40 Reps

45

Ask The Trainers

Prior to writing this book, I polled some friends online about questions they would love to have answered by a trainer. So this section consists of answers to FAQ by myself and other professional trainers.

1) What are some effective ways to get more energy?

First, make sure you are getting at least 7 hours of sleep. Secondly, take in more life giving foods such as fruits and XX, or XX for breakfast and also throughout the day. Thirdly, make sure that you are hydrated. Dehydration is king of making you sluggish and drowsy. I also believe that taking a good multivitamin is beneficial.

Lastly, I would suggest you make sure all electronics are off and away from your head when preparing for bed.

Chris Harrison
Owner CrossFit3816/Kingdom Athletics
Certified Personal Trainer
CrossFit Level I/II
USAW Level I

2) What is the best way to get micronutrients?

The best way is to eat VEGGIES. Pound the veggies and fruits. Personally, I don't like eating raw veggies, so I use a veggie mix drink that I can mix with water or juice. Also, a handful of spinach sautéed down to nothing is also easy to add to almost any meal. Find the veggies you like —so you won't feel disgusted by eating them—and then prepare them in a healthy way.

Donald Ezell, CPT
Fitness Trainer
Co-Owner of Iron Wolves Fitness

3) What is intermittent fasting?

Intermittent fasting or I.F., is a term that refers to cycling fasting periods within periods of eating. A more common cycle is to fast for 16 hours followed by an 8-hour eating window. This type of nutrition protocol is often used for the goal of fat loss.

I.F. has many benefits including fat accessibility as energy, by way of reducing insulin levels. This would also prevent type 2 diabetes. Plus, it helps reduce inflammation in the body while promoting cellular repair.

While the research is still pending on this, some reports suggest that it is possible that IF can help aid in the prevention of cancer and greater longevity.

Stephen Mass
B.S. Exercise Science
IFBB Professional

4) What are Repetitions (Reps)?

Repetitions, or reps for short, is one correctly completed full range of motion activity, or movement during an exercise.

Robert L. Wagner, CPT
Founder, Fit Christians

5) What are BCAAs?

Branch Chain Amino Acids (BCAAs) are: Leucine,

Isoleucine, and Valine. These amino acids are essential for muscle growth, performance boost, and improved workouts. Each of these have additional benefits, such as muscle protein synthesis (Leucine), fat loss and energy boost (Isoleucine) and minimized fatigued along with fat loss and prolonged energy (Valine). When I was preparing for competitions, my coach had me drinking 2 scoops of BCAAs mixed with 8oz of water mid-workout.

Robert L. Wagner, CPT
Founder, Fit Christians

6) How do you lose belly fat?

First, it's all about diet and changing the amount of calories intake and type of calories you're consuming Take in more protein, stabilize your carb intake (focusing more on slow digesting carbs, fibers and leafy foods). Also eat healthy fats to help retrain the body on metabolizing fat, and more omega 3s in a good rotation with omega 6s. Secondly, lifting heavier weight but making sure you maintain control of the weight. This inspires more fat-burning over a longer period of time. Bookend workouts with slow and steady cardio for 20+ minutes also helps.

Lovey Chuhtha
Founder, Lovey Fitness

7) Are there any alternatives to getting muscles warned up without stretching?

Jumping rope on a padded surface is the next best thing to stretching

Kendrick "The Apostle" Releford, CPT, Certified Boxing Coach
P.A.L. Boxing Coach
Co-Founder of Dream Performance Academy

8) Should I do cardio first or weight training first?

My first response to this question is: what is cardio? There's a great misconception about what cardio actually is. Most people hop on a treadmill to try and run off fat to get in shape. So they're equating cardio with a treadmill, almost exclusively. Even worst, they believe that weight training will make them bigger.

Here's the truth. Cardio has everything to do with your cardiovascular system. In short, it's about getting the blood pumping in your heart. The more intensely it pumps blood through the body the more cardio at work.

So the fact is, cardio happens during weight training as well as cycling, aerobic training or treadmill. Whether one uses body weight, weight lifting or a combination of both (which I prefer) cardio is happening. What's better in my opinion is that you're developing strength and building muscle, which enables you to burn more fat while at rest. It won't make you bulky, in fact for me I got smaller through weight training.

What I'd suggest is that you monitor your time in between reps during a workout. You can also track your heart rate. To test this theory, try a workout that includes burpees or pushups and watch how forcefully your cardio kicks in. Add to the end of your workout 10 rounds of 30-second sprints with 20-second breaks if you really want some form of running; the more intensity the better.

If your goal is to look like a marathon runner, then by all means...hop on a track and run. If you want to look like a sprinter, short bursts of speed and weight training are the way to go.

Lastly, if you're overweight as I was, look around the room. Take a look at those who you'd truly want your body to look like. What you'll notice is, for the most part, is that they're all weight training! You burn more fat in the long run through intense weight training and healthy eating. Running may seem more productive, but in some cases it may burn more muscle, and though you're getting smaller you're not getting stronger & worst, the fats are not going away. Train with and like those you want to be like.

Sean Reed
Personal Trainer

9) What is peak week?

It is the week preceding the major event after weeks, months or years of eating clean and lifting weights. It is the final week of touches leading up to the event. It can also be the week leading up to summer trip, or a photo shoot. Now peak week is only optimal if you are around single digits in body fat, although it can add value wherever you are. Here is a common daily list of things to do for a successful peak week.

* Days 1-3: Low or no carbs, super high water and sodium intake, and high rep workouts to help in depletion.
* Days 4 & 5: Aggressively start carb load and by Thursday begin reducing sodium and water intake. Also, cease workouts beginning Wednesday.
* Day 6: Continue carb loading and water reduction. Also, a nice diuretic supplement or natural one (i.e. Asparagus.
* Day 7: Continue to load on carbs and consume no water. It would also help consuming potassium to prevent cramping.

There are different ways to engage a Peak Week, and each person's body responds differently. In my experience, the more I enter Peak Week, the more I learn about my body and what to do or not do.

Robert L. Wagner, CPT
Founder, Fit Christians

10) Do you have any Gym Etiquette tips?

- 1) No Texting

Have you ever been to the gym to find someone hogging the bench? They are not lifting, but rather sitting and texting. The next time you have the need to text, jump off the machine and let it serve its purpose.

- 2) Shower First

Showering before your gym time actually has some benefits. It can raise your body temperature, kickstart blood flow, and get your muscles loosen for the workout ahead. Also, There there is nothing worse than distracting others with your smell. So help others and clean up a bit.

- 3) Come Prepared

Many times people in the gym are confused about what they want to actually do. They bounce from machine to machine or just come take a picture and leave because they are overwhelmed. Always have a plan of action!

- 4) Check Before You Wreck

Before sitting down and taking over a machine, look around and ask the nearest person, "Are you working out on this machine?" It's always polite to make sure someone isn't in the midst of their sets or doing a superset.

- 5) Bring A Towel

If you are one of those super sweaty people, bring yourself a towel to protect the rest of the world from all of your sweat. There is nothing worse than approaching a gym and seeing sweat bubbles on the bench. A microfiber towel is a great choice.

Robert L. Wagner, CPT
Founder, Fit Christians

46

10 Things To Put Wings On Your Dreams

As this book comes to a close, I want to thank you for taking the time to read and interact and support it. I hope and pray you were encouraged in your fitness journey. As a kid, I once read the poem *Dream Deferred* by Langston Hughes and it had me wondering a lot about what happens to dreams. Like really, what happens to them? Do they really dry up, or maybe sag. Needless to say, I don't want my dreams to be deferred. It's my desire that the dreams you and I have will take off and become a reality. –And with that, below are 10 priorities you need to consider to put wings on your dreams:

Prayer – God honors our dependence upon Him, therefore spend time saturating your thoughts and dreams in prayer. In spending time with Him, our desires are literally affected by His. In essence, His desires become our dreams.

Picture It – Oftentimes, we spend too much of our energy focusing on the things we don't want to do. How about utilizing that same energy to focus on what you want to do instead?

Positivity – All things begin with a willing mind. Change your perspective on how you see things and watch how it opens the flow of your productivity.

Planning – Preparation enhances your chances for success. If Jesus tells us to count up the cost (Luke 14:25-33), then proper preparation prevents poor performance.

Persistence – Talent is what you are born with, but skills are what you spend hours perfecting. Many people are talented but they lack in the proper skills. I encourage you to be consistent about spending time perfecting your craft and watch how your gifts make room for you.

Promoting – Learn how to articulate and sell yourself without being overbearing or cocky. In order for people to see the greatness you have, you must put yourself in a position to be seen. *"No one lights a lamp and then puts it under a basket, a lamp is placed on a stand, where it gives light to everyone in the house"* (Matt. 5:15). What value will you bring your generation and the next if no one knows who you are or what you can offer?

Playtime – Find time to enjoy the fruit of your labors along the way. Enjoy your Reward Meals. Again, these meals allow you the opportunity to avoid potential pitfalls and burn out. In the same manner, we should enjoy the fruits of our labor to help avoid burn out.

Patience – It takes time for your dreams to come to past, therefore remain patient and committed to endurance. *Remember those that wait on the Lord will renew their strength (Is. 40:31).*

Praise – Praise God along the way that your dream is already fulfilled. We should also be sure to praise others and not overly criticize those who help us along the way.

Pride – If nobody else does, make sure you believe in you. God has uniquely gifted each of us with what we need, in order to do what He has called us to do. Be proud of who you are and remember, "no one can do what you do like you do it."

What are your dreams? How can we pray for you?

prayer@wakepraytrain.com

47

Join The Conversation

WEBSITE: ROBERTLWAGNER.COM

FACEBOOK: @ROBERTLWAGNER07

TWITTER: @ROBERTLWAGNER

YOUTUBE: @ROBERTLWAGNER

VISIT HTTP://WAKEPRAYTRAIN.COM FOR
SHIRTS, TANKS, AND OTHER ACCESSORIES.
REP YOUR FAITH IN THE GYM OR EVERY DAY.

#WAKEPRAYTRAIN #FITCHRISTIANS
#GLORIFYGODWITHYOURFITNESS

About Robert L. Wagner

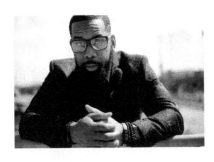

A bible teacher, trainer, speaker, and media personality. Robert wrote his first book entitled Conversations: Developing An Intimate Dialogue With God in 2014. Robert has an extreme passion to see people grow spiritually, naturally and physically as seen by his 20+ years of experience as a 'trainer. One of his generation's most creative bible expositors delivering high energy, creativity and in-depth instruction to each presentation. He is a graduate of Dallas Theological Seminary and is motivated by the vision for his life which is to "bring life to dead places."

CPSIA information can be obtained
at www.ICGtesting.com
Printed in the USA
LVHW050726181020
668893LV00003B/289

9 780692 135716